THIS BOOK IS FOR YOU

You recently may have been told that you have diabetes. If so, this book will help you understand and manage your disease.

If you have had diabetes for a while and have experienced a change in health, or if you are having trouble controlling your blood sugar, your doctor may have started you on diabetes pills or insulin injections.

In either case, you may be feeling scared, angry, overwhelmed, or possibly even guilty about your current health condition. These feelings are normal. You may find that sharing your feelings with your friends and loved ones will help you work through them. Everyone has low days. People with diabetes are no different. If your feelings start getting in the way of taking care of yourself, talk to someone.

There is no cure for diabetes, but with the help of your health care team, you can treat your diabetes, take charge of it, and manage it.

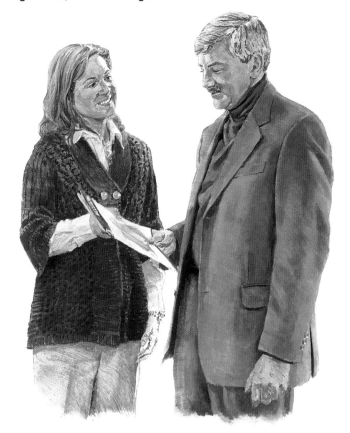

WHAT IS DIABETES?

When you have diabetes, the food you eat cannot be used for energy because your body is not making enough of the hormone, **insulin**, OR the insulin you have is not working the way it should. Insulin is made in the pancreas, an organ that lies behind the stomach.

Here's how insulin normally works:

Most food is broken down into a form of sugar called glucose. Sugar is the body's main source of energy. As sugar enters the bloodstream, the amount of sugar in the blood rises. Normally the body reacts to the rise in blood sugar by signaling the pancreas to send insulin into the bloodstream.

Insulin helps sugar leave the bloodstream and enter the cells. To understand how insulin works, think of a cell as a house with many locked doors. Insulin is the key that unlocks the doors and lets sugar leave the bloodstream and enter the cells. **Wherever insulin travels in the body, it opens up the cells so sugar can enter them.** After sugar gets into the body's cells, the cells can immediately use it for energy or store it for use later on.

Here's what happens when you have diabetes:

Your pancreas makes little or no insulin OR the insulin you have is not working the way it should. Either way, sugar cannot get into your body's cells. Instead of entering the cells, it stays trapped in the bloodstream, raising the amount of sugar in your blood to abnormally high levels.

Your kidneys get rid of some of the extra sugar by filtering it from your blood and removing it from your body through your urine. But your blood sugar is still too high.

Cell

Sugar (glucose)

Insulin

Bloodstream

2

SIGNS OF DIABETES

Because your body is not getting the sugar it needs, you are likely to feel tired. You may urinate more often than usual, you may be very thirsty, or you may lose weight even though you are eating the way you normally do. These are all signs of diabetes.

Unfortunately, your body cannot lower blood sugar by itself. You have to help. You can do this by balancing what you eat with regular exercise, medications (if prescribed), and weight loss (if you are overweight). You can learn to control your diabetes so it doesn't control you. Controlling diabetes means keeping your blood sugar as close to normal as possible—not too high and not too low.

What is a normal blood sugar range?

According to the *American Diabetes Association,* a normal *fasting* blood sugar range for a person who does not have diabetes is less than 100 mg/dL.

A **target blood sugar range** is a range that most people with diabetes should try to achieve. When blood sugar is less than 70 mg/dL, most people feel the symptoms of low blood sugar. Research shows that when blood sugars are greater than 150 mg/dL, the risk for complications increases.

The target blood sugar for most people with diabetes is 90 to 130 mg/dL before meals. This target range may be different for people who do not feel the symptoms of low blood sugar; people with serious medical problems; elderly people or very young people (under the age of puberty); and women who are pregnant.

Your health care team will determine your target blood sugar range. You may be asked to test your blood sugar before you eat meals and/or two hours after you eat a meal. Testing at different times of the day helps your health care team determine if you need medication for diabetes or if you have the right diabetes medication.

TYPES OF DIABETES

A breakdown in how your body uses sugar (glucose) for energy can lead to two major types of diabetes: Type 1 and Type 2.

TYPE 1 DIABETES

With Type 1 diabetes, the body makes little or no insulin on its own. People with Type 1 diabetes need two or more insulin shots each day. About 1 in 10 people with diabetes have Type 1. It can develop in older adults, but it often occurs in a child, adolescent, or young adult.

Signs of Type 1 diabetes:

- frequent urination
- increased thirst
- lack or increase in appetite
- rapid weight loss (even when eating normally)
- dizziness
- very dry or itchy skin
- fatigue
- blurred vision

The symptoms may come on suddenly, but experts believe Type 1 diabetes actually develops over a long period of time.

Causes of Type 1 diabetes:

- There may be a history of diabetes in the family.

- A virus may injure the pancreas, reducing its ability to make insulin.

- The body's immune system may mistakenly destroy the insulin-producing cells in the pancreas.

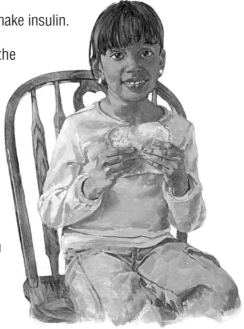

To manage Type 1 diabetes:

- **Monitor your blood sugar.** Self-monitoring (checking) your blood sugar is the best way to know how well your diabetes is being managed.

- **Take insulin every day.** Since your body is making little if any insulin, you need daily insulin shots.

- **Follow a meal plan.** A meal plan will help you eat the right kinds and amounts of food.

- **Exercise.** Balancing exercise with the food you eat and the insulin you take will help keep your blood sugar within your target range.

TYPE 2 DIABETES

Most people with diabetes have Type 2. With this type, the body usually makes insulin, but the insulin does not work the way it should. Sometimes, the body does not make enough insulin. Type 2 diabetes tends to occur in older adults. However, a growing number of children and adolescents are now developing Type 2 diabetes.

Signs of Type 2 diabetes:

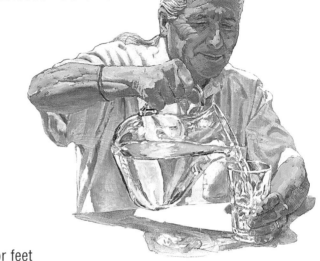

- frequent urination
- fatigue
- increased thirst
- very dry or itchy skin
- sores that are slow to heal
- unexplained weight loss
- extreme hunger
- sudden vision change
- tingling or numbness in the hands or feet

The symptoms usually develop over a long period of time. Some people with Type 2 diabetes have mild symptoms or no symptoms at all.

Generally, children at risk:

- have a family history of Type 2 diabetes
- are overweight or obese
- are physically inactive
- belong to a high-risk ethnic or racial group (such as Native American, African-American, Hispanic-American, Asian-American, or Pacific Islander)

Generally, adults at risk:

While the exact cause is not known, Type 2 diabetes is more likely to occur in high-risk people, such as those who:

- are over 45 years old
- are overweight or obese
- have a history of gestational diabetes (or women who have delivered a large baby - greater than 9 pounds)
- are physically inactive
- belong to a high-risk ethnic or racial group (such as Native American, African-American, Hispanic-American, Asian-American, or Pacific Islander)

TO MANAGE TYPE 2 DIABETES:

- **Monitor your blood sugar.** Self-monitoring (checking) of your blood sugar is one of the best ways of knowing how well your diabetes is being managed.

- **Follow a meal plan.** A meal plan will help you eat the right kinds and amounts of food.

- **Exercise regularly.** Regular exercise helps you make better use of your own insulin.

- **Maintain a healthy weight.** Many people with Type 2 diabetes are overweight. Being overweight puts a person at risk for developing Type 2 diabetes.

  Sugar gets into the cells through special doors called receptor sites. An overweight person has fewer receptor sites. Losing weight can increase the number of receptor sites and may lower blood sugar. Weight loss may be one of the most important factors in helping control blood sugar in overweight people with Type 2 diabetes.

- **Take medication** (if needed). Not everyone with Type 2 diabetes needs medication. Following a meal plan and exercising regularly may control your blood sugar. If this doesn't work, a pill may be prescribed to help your body make more insulin or make better use of the insulin you have.

  If pills do not lower your blood sugar enough, insulin injections or other injectable medications may be needed to help control your blood sugar.

  If you have questions about your treatment program, talk to your doctor, diabetes nurse, or diabetes educator.

Never take more or less medication than the amount prescribed.

YOUR TREATMENT PROGRAM

Your treatment program will involve a meal plan, an exercise plan, and medication (if needed). Managing your diabetes may involve working with a team of health care professionals, such as your:

- doctor
- certified diabetes educator
- registered dietitian

- pharmacist
- ophthalmologist (eye doctor)
- podiatrist (foot doctor)

Your meal plan

Learning how to eat well is an essential part of managing diabetes. The right foods can help you keep your weight healthy and your blood sugar at a steady level. Eating well is the key to taking control of your diabetes and avoiding diabetes-related problems. Begin with these guidelines:

- Eat 3 balanced meals a day.
- Eat at the same time each day.
- Eat meals 4 to 5 hours apart.

- Avoid high-sugar foods.
- Avoid high-sugar drinks.
- Include a bedtime snack.

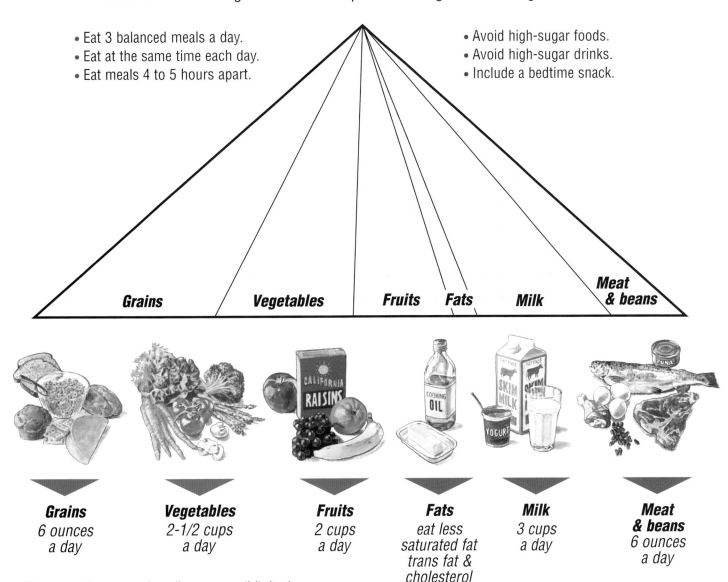

Grains
6 ounces
a day

Vegetables
2-1/2 cups
a day

Fruits
2 cups
a day

Fats
eat less
saturated fat
trans fat &
cholesterol

Milk
3 cups
a day

**Meat
& beans**
6 ounces
a day

These amounts may vary depending on your activity level.

FOOD CONTAINS 3 KINDS OF NUTRIENTS:

- carbohydrates
- protein
- fat

 Make sure you eat foods from each of these food groups.

Carbohydrates affect blood sugar the most. They are the body's main source of energy. Carbohydrate choices include bread, cereal, pasta; starchy vegetables, like potatoes or corn; dried beans, lentils, rice; fruits and fruit juices; milk, yogurt, and other dairy foods; sweets, like cookies, candy, regular soda pop, sugar, and syrup.

About 90 to 100% of the carbohydrates you eat enter your blood within a couple of hours after you eat them. Proteins and fats are slower to digest and do not affect blood sugar as rapidly as carbohydrates do.

Counting carbohydrates

The total number of carbohydrates you should eat at a meal or snack is based on your weight, age, activity level, and eating habits. A dietitian can help you decide the number of carbohydrates you need.

When you count carbohydrates, you keep track of foods that contain carbohydrates. A serving of any food from a carbohydrate group is considered to be equal. All carbohydrates are treated as a single group in which trade-offs are possible.

One serving of bread has the same carbohydrate value as 1 serving of fruit. One serving of potato has the same carbohydrate value as 1 serving of milk. **One (1) serving or choice equals 15 grams of carbohydrate.**

You can count carbohydrate **grams**, or you can count carbohydrate **choices** *or* **servings**. You prefer to think in terms of carbohydrate choices or servings instead of grams. Using this system does not mean you have to eat the same things every day—you simply need to eat similar types of food.

WHAT IS A CHOICE OR SERVING?

A choice or serving can be determined by reading the nutrition label on a food package or looking at published food lists.

The nutrition label tells the serving size and how much carbohydrate the serving contains. Remember the number 15. **A carbohydrate choice or serving is equal to 15 grams of carbohydrate.** The following pages contain lists (or examples) of carbohydrates. Each food listed also has a serving size. Here are examples of serving sizes.

1 carbohydrate choice (15 grams of carbohydrate)	2 carbohydrate choices (30 grams of carbohydrate)	3 carbohydrate choices (45 grams of carbohydrate)
1 slice of bread	2 slices of bread	2 slices of bread and 1 cup of yogurt
1/3 cup cooked pasta	2/3 cup cooked pasta	1 cup cooked pasta
1 small piece of fruit	1 large piece of fruit	1 1/2 cups flaked cereal and 1 cup of milk

Below is a general guide for planning a balanced meal. Your dietitian will work with you to develop a meal plan that meets your individual needs.

	Inactive women	Women	Inactive men	Men
Carbohydrate per meal	30-45 grams (2-3 carb choices)	45-60 grams (3-4 carb choices)	45-60 grams (3-4 carb choices)	60-75 grams (4-5 carb choices)
Protein per meal	2 oz.	2-3 oz.	2-3 oz.	3-4 oz.
Servings added **Fat** per meal	1	1-2	1-2	2-3
Calories per day	1200-1400	1500-1800	1500-1800	2000-2400
Carbohydrate per day	150 gm	200 gm	200 gm	300 gm

Selecting healthy foods and planning when you eat can help you feel better and achieve good diabetes control. Discuss any questions or concerns you may have with your dietitian or your diabetes educator.

CARBOHYDRATE CHOICES

The lists that appear on pages 10 through 14 are examples of only a few foods. Talk to your dietitian if you would like more information.

STARCH

(1 choice = 15 grams of carbohydrate and 80 calories)

Bread

White or wheat bread	1 slice (1 oz.)
Bagel, large (4 oz.)	1/4
English muffin	1/2 (1 oz.)
French toast	1 slice
Hamburger bun	1/2 (1 oz.)
Muffin, low-fat	1 small
Pita pocket - 6 inch	1/2
Pancake, from mix - 4 inch	1
Tortilla, corn - 6 inch	1
Tortilla, flour - 6 inch	1
Waffle, 4 1/2 inch	1

Cereal

Bran cereal	1/2 cup
Corn flakes	3/4 cup
Granola, low-fat	1/4 cup
Grape Nuts®	1/4 cup
Hot cereal, like	
Cream of Wheat	1/2 cup
Oatmeal - old fashioned	1/2 cup
Oatmeal - instant	1 package
Puffed cereal	1 1/2 cup
Raisin bran	1/3 cup
Sugar frosted cereal	1/2 cup

Crackers and snacks

Animal crackers	8
Graham crackers	3 squares
Pretzels	3/4 oz.
Saltine-type crackers	6
Popcorn, no fat added	3 cups

Pasta and grains

Cornmeal (dry)	3 Tbsp.
Cornstarch (dry)	2 Tbsp.
Pasta, cooked	1/3 cup
Rice, white (cooked)	1/3 cup
Rice, brown (cooked)	1/3 cup

Starchy vegetables

Canned beans (pinto, navy, kidney)	1/2 cup
Baked beans	1/3 cup
Corn, canned	1/2 cup
Corn on the cob	1 medium ear
Peas, green	1/2 cup

Starchy vegetables

Potato, baked or boiled	1 small
Potato, mashed	1/2 cup
Squash	1 cup
Yam	1/2 cup
Sweet potato	1/2 cup

FRUIT

(1 choice = 15 grams of carbohydrate and 60 calories)

Apple, unpeeled	1 small
Banana - 4 inch	1
Blueberries, blackberries	3/4 cup
Canned fruit, unsweetened	1/2 cup
Grapefruit	1/2 large
Grapes or cherries	12 to 15
Orange	1 small
Raisins	2 Tbsp.

Raspberries	1 cup
Strawberries, fresh	1 1/4 cup
Watermelon	1 cup

Fruit juice

Apple, orange	1/2 cup (4 oz.)
Grapefruit, pineapple	1/2 cup (4 oz.)
Grape, peach, pear, prune	1/3 cup (3 oz.)
Cranberry juice, reduced cal.	1 cup (8 oz.)

MILK

(1 choice = 12-15 grams of carbohydrate and 90 to 150 calories)

Whole, 1% or 2% milk	1 cup	Yogurt, fruit-flavored, nonfat or	
Skim or lowfat milk	1 cup	low-fat, artificially sweetened	1 cup
Yogurt, fruit-flavored, light	1 cup	Buttermilk, nonfat or low-fat	1 cup

OTHER CARBOHYDRATE CHOICES

These foods can fit into your meal plan, but the serving sizes are smaller and they lack important vitamins and minerals. (1 choice = 15 grams of carbohydrate)

Brownie, unfrosted - 2-inch square	1	Ice cream, regular or light	1/2 cup
Cake, no icing - 2-inch square	1 piece	Jam, jelly, honey, syrup, regular	1 Tbsp.
Casserole	1/2 cup	Jelly beans	9
Chocolate syrup	2 Tbsp.	LifeSavers®	8
Cocoa mix, sugar-free, reduced cal.	3 Tbsp.	Pudding, no sugar,	
Cookie, with cream filling	2 small	made w/skim milk	1/2 cup
Cookie, sugar-free	3 small	Pie, pumpkin or custard	1/16 of pie
Frozen yogurt, nonfat or low-fat	1/3 cup	Pizza, thin crust	1 slice
Frozen yogurt, fat-free, sugar-free	1/2 cup	Potato chips	12-18 chips
Frozen fruit juice bars, 100% juice	1 bar	Tortilla chips	9-13 chips
Gatorade®	1 cup	Salad dressing, fat-free	1/4 cup
Gelatin, regular	1/2 cup	Sherbet or sorbet	1/4 cup
Gingersnaps	3	Soup (most kinds)	1 cup
Granola bar	1 bar	Spaghetti sauce	1/2 cup

NON-STARCHY VEGETABLES

(1 choice = 5 grams of carbohydrate and 25 calories)

A choice or **serving is 1/2 cup of cooked vegetables or 1 cup of raw vegetables**. You should eat 3 to 5 servings of vegetables a day. A serving of vegetables at meal or snack time does not have to be counted in your meal plan.

Artichokes	Cabbage	Kohlrabi	Radishes
Asparagus	Carrots	Leeks	Salad greens
Beans (green, wax)	Cauliflower	Mushrooms	Spinach
Bean sprouts	Celery	Okra	Tomatoes
Beets	Cucumbers	Onions	Turnips
Broccoli	Eggplant	Pea pods	Water chestnuts
Brussel sprouts	Green onions	Peppers	Zucchini

Since these vegetables are high in nutrients and lower in calories they do not affect your blood sugar as much as starchy vegetables, such as corn and peas.

Choose different colored vegetables - green, yellow, orange, white, red and purple.

PROTEIN

Protein is one of the three major sources of calories in your diet. Protein provides nutrients for building cells, tissue, bones, and muscles. **A serving of protein is 1 ounce. Two to 3 ounces of protein are usually suggested at each meal.** Your dietitian will tell you how much protein to eat. Meat servings are based on cooked meats with fat and bone removed. Meat can have a lot of fat - a serving may contain 3 to 8 grams of fat. When possible, buy lean meats and low-fat or fat-free cheeses and other foods.

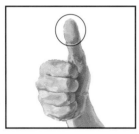

The thumb to the first joint represents 1 ounce

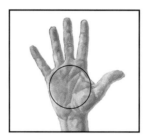

The palm of a woman's hand is about 3 ounces

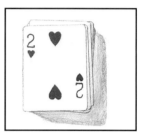

A deck of cards represents about 3 ounces

MEAT AND MEAT SUBSTITUTES (PROTEIN)

(1 choice = 0 gms of carbohydrate, 7 gms of protein, and 3-8 gms of fat and 50-100 calories)

Meat (1 ounce portion)		Meat substitutes	
Beef	Turkey	Cottage cheese	1/4 cup
Chicken	Veal	Cheese	1 oz.
Fish	Seafood	Egg	1
Lamb		Nuts	1/4 cup
Pork		Peanut butter	1 Tbsp.
Wild game		Tofu	1/2 cup

FAT CHOICES

(1 choice = 0 gms of carbohydrate, 5 gms of fat and 45 calories)

Oil (canola, olive, peanut, etc.)	1 tsp.	Butter	1 tsp.
Margarine, reduced-fat	1 Tbsp.	Cream, half and half	2 Tbsp.
Mayonnaise	1 tsp.	Nuts, almonds, cashews	6 nuts
Mayonnaise, reduced-fat	1 Tbsp.	Peanuts	10 nuts
Salad dressing, reduced-fat	2 Tbsp.	Peanut butter	1 tsp.
Cream cheese	1 Tbsp.	Shortening	1 tsp.
Cream cheese, reduced-fat	2 Tbsp.	Sour cream	2 Tbsp.
Cheese sauce	2 Tbsp.	Sour cream, reduced-fat	3 Tbsp.

Fats are the most concentrated source of calories. Your body needs some fat. It is only when you eat too much fat or the wrong kind of fat that it becomes a problem.

MORE ABOUT FAT

Saturated fats are found mainly in foods that come from animals. They are hard at room temperature. Eating too much fat, especially saturated fat, can lead to high cholesterol. Having high cholesterol increases your risk of cardiovascular disease (heart attack or stroke).

Trans fats also can increase your risk of cardiovascular disease. Trans fats are created by adding hydrogen to vegetable oils during a process called hydrogenation. Trans fats may be found in commercially baked goods, stick margarine, and vegetable shortening, *and* they are often used to fry foods.

Unsaturated fats mainly come from plants. They can be monounsaturated or polyunsaturated. These fats are usually liquid at room temperature. Polyunsaturated and monounsaturated fats are high in total fat and have as many calories as saturated fat. Ask your dietitian for advice on including these fats in your diet.

Omega-3 fatty acids are fats which seem to positively influence a number of factors related to protection from cardio-vascular disease. Your dietitian may suggest that you add or eat more foods which contain Omega-3 fats.

To reduce the fat in your meals:

- **Choose lean meat.** Avoid high-fat meat choices, such as luncheon meats or hot dogs. Limit high-fat choices to 3 times (or less) a week.

- **Trim the fat from meat and remove the skin from poultry** (like chicken or turkey) before cooking. Bake, broil, grill, or steam foods instead of frying.

- **Include low-fat or nonfat foods in your meal plan.** For example, use fat-free or low-fat cheese and yogurt rather than the regular versions. Replace regular salad dressings with low-fat or nonfat dressings.

- **Use vegetable oils whenever possible** in baking and cooking. Often 3/4 cup of liquid oil may be used in place of 1 cup of solid shortening.

Fat can be saturated, polyunsaturated, monounsaturated or a mixture of these fats.

No more than 25 to 35% of your total daily calories should come from fat.

Foods that are high in saturated fat:
bacon
butter & lard
sausage (all kinds)
polish dogs & hot dogs
luncheon meats
solid shortening
potato & corn chips
cream & sour cream
ice cream
chocolate
fat in red meat
poultry skin
cocoa butter
coconut & palm oil
regular cheese
whole-milk dairy products
fried foods

Trans fats
baked goods
fried foods
solid shortening
French fries
doughnuts & cookies
stick margarine

Polyunsaturated fats
corn oil, safflower oil
sesame oil, soybean oil
sunflower oil & seeds

Monounsaturated fats
avocados
canola, olive & peanut oil
most nuts

Omega-3 fats
fish oil, flax oil, canola oil
fish, such as herring,
  mackerel, salmon
English walnuts,
  butternuts, soybeans
flax seed (ground)

FREE FOODS

Any food or drink that contains less than 5 grams of carbohydrate per serving can be counted as a "free food." Foods listed with a serving size, but less than 5 grams of carbohydrate, should be limited to 3 servings a day. These foods must be spread throughout the day. If you eat all 3 servings at one time, you will have to count the food as a carbohydrate serving. Here are some examples of free foods:

FAT-FREE OR REDUCED-FAT

Cream cheese, fat-free	1 Tbsp.
Cocoa powder, unsweetened	1 Tbsp.
Non-dairy creamer (liquid)	1 Tbsp.
Non-dairy creamer (powder)	2 tsp.
Mayonnaise, fat-free	1 Tbsp.
Mayonnaise, reduced-fat	1 tsp.
Miracle Whip®, fat-free	1 Tbsp.
Miracle Whip®, reduced-fat	1 tsp.
Margarine, fat-free	4 Tbsp.
Margarine, reduced-fat	1 tsp.
Salad dressing, fat-free	1 Tbsp.
Whipped topping (like Cool Whip®)	2 Tbsp.
Salsa	1/4 cup
Sour cream, fat-free or low-fat	1 Tbsp.
Yogurt, fat-free	2 Tbsp.

CONDIMENTS

Barbecue sauce	1 Tbsp.
Butter Buds®	3 tsp.
Catsup	1 Tbsp.
Chili sauce	1 Tbsp.
Cocktail sauce	1 Tbsp.
Dill pickle - large	1 1/2
Horseradish	3 Tbsp.
Molly McButter®	2 tsp.
Mrs. Dash®	1 tsp.
Mustard	1 Tbsp.
Picante sauce	2 Tbsp.
Soy sauce	1 Tbsp.
Steak sauce	1 Tbsp.
Taco sauce	1 Tbsp.
Worcestershire sauce	1 Tbsp.

SEASONINGS

Garlic
Herbs (basil, oregano, rosemary, thyme, etc.)
Lemon juice
Lime juice
Pimento
Spices
Flavoring extracts
Cooking wine
Cooking spray
Vinegar

BEVERAGES (DRINKS)

Beef broth	1 cup
Chicken broth	1/2 cup
Carbonated water	
Club soda	
Coffee (without sugar)	
Diet soda	
Kool-aid® (sugar-free)	
Mineral water	
Tang® (sugar-free)	
Tea (without sugar)	
Sugar-free drink mixes	

SUGAR-FREE OR LOW-SUGAR

Sugar-free hard candy	1 piece
Sugar-free gelatin	
Sugar-free popsicles	
Sugar-free gum	
Sugar-free jam or jelly	
Jam or jelly, low-sugar	2 Tbsp.
Sugar-free syrup	
Sugar substitutes, like	
Equal® (aspartame)	
Sweet'n Low, Sugar Twin (saccharin)	
Splenda®, Sweet One (acesulfame K)	

READING LABELS

The Nutrition Facts label will tell you how much carbohydrate, protein, fat, cholesterol, sugar, sodium, and calories are in 1 serving.

Check the serving size. It may be less than the amount you are likely to eat. If you only look at the total carbohydrates, the food may fit into your meal plan. But once you compare serving size and total carbohydrates, you may only be able to eat a very small amount of the food.

Check the total carbohydrate in 1 serving. Sugars are part of the total carbohydrate listed on the label. This macaroni and cheese meal contains 31 grams of carbohydrate or 2 carbohydrate choices.

Pay attention to how much total fat the food contains. You should have no more than 50 to 60 grams of total fat per day. **Pay attention to how much saturated fat and trans fat the food contains**. No more than 7% of your total daily calories should come from saturated fat. Generally, that amount is between 15 and 20 grams of saturated fat or trans fat per day. Check the amount of cholesterol the food contains. You should have no more than 200 milligrams of cholesterol a day.

Check the amount of sodium the food contains. You should have no more than 2000 to 2400 milligrams of sodium a day (or less depending on your doctor's advice).

A common recommendation for fiber is 20 to 35 grams a day. Ask your dietitian how much fiber you should have.

The label on this page was taken from a can of chili with beans. This is only a sample label. This food may not be a good choice for you. Ask your dietitian for advice.

Nutrition Facts

Serving Size 1 cup (247g)
Servings Per Container 2

Amount Per Serving

Calories 260   Calories from fat 60

	% Daily Value *
Total Fat 7g	11%
Saturated Fat 3g	15%
Trans Fat 2g	
Cholesterol 30mg	10%
Sodium 1200mg	50%
Total Carbohydrate 33g	11%
Dietary Fiber 7g	28%
Sugars 5g	
Protein 16g	

Vitamin A	10%	Vitamin C	0%
Calcium	6%	Iron	15%

* Percent Daily Values are based on a 2,000 calorie diet. Your daily values may be higher or lower depending on your calorie needs.

Carbohydrate choices	Grams of carbohydrate
1	11 – 20
1-1/2	21 – 25
2	26 – 35
2-1/2	36 – 40
3	41 – 50
3-1/2	51 – 55
4	56 – 65
4-1/2	66 – 70
5	71 – 80

JUICY
1 small orange or apple
1 cup watermelon
1-1/4 cup strawberries
3/4 cup peaches or
  pineapple
1 cup honeydew
1 medium kiwi
Canned:
1/2 cup peaches in juice
1/2 cup pears in juice

SALTY
Chips
  10-12 any flavor
Pretzels:
8 regular
12 mini or sticks
Crackers:
45 Goldfish®
40 Ritz Bits®
27 Cheez-Its®
19 Cheese Nips®,
  reduced-fat
24 Cheese Nips®, regular
12 Wheat Thins®
3 Triscuits®, reduced-fat
5 Triscuits®, regular
3 cups of popcorn

CRUNCHY
Cookies:
16 Teddy Grahams®
6 vanilla wafers
3 gingersnaps
2 Chips Ahoy®
2 Nutter Butter®
2 E.L. Fudge®
1 oatmeal raisin
1 rice krispie treat

SMOOTH
1/2 medium banana
1/2 c. sugar-free pudding
1/2 c. unsweetened
  applesauce
1 Lite yogurt, any flavor
1/2 c. frozen yogurt,
  sugar-free
1 fudge bar, sugar-free

SNACK IDEAS

You can satisfy your cravings and follow your meal plan with these snack ideas. **The amounts listed here are equal to 1 carbohydrate serving or 15 grams of carbohydrate.** Since the amounts may vary depending on the brands and size of the food item, it's a good idea to check the nutrition facts label for the amount of carbohydrates the food contains.

Snacks with protein:

- 1/2 of a sandwich

- 1/2 of an English muffin with peanut butter

- 6 whole-grain crackers and 1 piece of string cheese

- 3 graham cracker squares with 1-tablespoon peanut butter

- 3 cups popcorn with 1/4 cup nuts
  (except honey-roasted)

- 3/4 cup unsweetened ready to eat cereal with 1-cup 1% or skim milk

- 1/2 cup sugar-free ice cream with 1/4 cup of nuts
  (except honey-roasted)

- 9-13 tortilla chips with 1/4 cup salsa and 1 oz. cheddar sauce

- 2 rice cakes (4 inches across) or 1/4 bagel with 2-tablespoons fat-free cream cheese and 2 teaspoons sugar-free or light jam or jelly

- 1/2 cup lite canned fruit with 1/4 cup cottage cheese

- 6 ounces fat-free, sugar-free, fruit flavored yogurt with 1-tablespoon granola

- 8 animal crackers with 1-cup of 1% or skim milk

Some of these snack ideas may affect fasting blood sugar levels. If your fasting blood sugars are over your goal, try avoiding dairy products and fruit as an evening (bedtime) snack.

PORTION CONTROL

A big problem for people with diabetes, as well as the general population, is large portions of food. Knowing how much food to eat is just as important as knowing what kinds of food to eat. You can't use restaurant servings as a guide because so many of them are super-sized. In reality, a serving is small by comparison.

Being able to identify portion sizes will help you balance the amount of food you eat. At first you may need to measure serving sizes so you will know what 1/2 cup of cereal or 1 tablespoon of peanut butter looks like. Foods should be measured after they have been cooked and the fat and bones have been removed. These suggestions will help you remember what a serving size looks like.

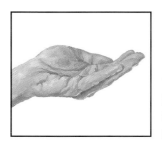

1 to 2 ounces is what a cupped hand can hold

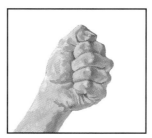

1 cup is equal to a fist

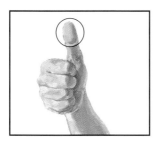

1 teaspoon is about the size of a thumb tip

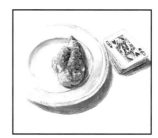

3 ounces of cooked chicken is the size of a deck of cards

It's easy to take a "little extra" or eat "a couple of bites." But it all adds up. Extra carbohydrates raise your blood sugar. Extra calories increase your weight. Check yourself every couple of months. Sit down to a usual meal but before eating, measure your servings. How close are you to the actual serving size?

Stay committed to your meal plan

Rather than giving up your plan because you overate at one or two meals, learn from your mistakes and try again. One or two setbacks should not stop your meal planning efforts.

MORE ABOUT THE FOOD YOU EAT

Artificial sweeteners

These sweeteners contain no sugar and few, if any, calories. They will not affect your blood sugar. There are also brown sugar artificial sweeteners that may be helpful in your meal planning. Some artificial sweeteners break down differently when used in cooking, and the cooked food may taste bitter. Read the label before you cook with these products. Artificial sweeteners are sweeter than table sugar, so less of the product is needed to sweeten foods.

Dietetic foods

These foods may not be calorie free or even lower in calories. Some have less sodium and/or sugar than regular foods, but they may be higher in fat. Some have fewer calories, but they may be higher in total carbohydrates. A product may have less sucrose (table sugar), but the sucrose may have been replaced with another form of sugar. **Check the label to see if the food is a good choice.**

Cholesterol

Cholesterol is a fat-like substance that circulates through your body in your blood. Most cholesterol is made by your body. The rest of it comes from the foods you eat. Cholesterol is found in foods that come from animals, like shellfish, organ meats, and egg yolks. You need a certain amount of cholesterol for normal body function. But having too much cholesterol in your blood increases your risk for a heart attack or stroke. **Limit these high-cholesterol foods.**

Sodium

Sodium is found naturally in many foods. It is added to foods during processing and is found in higher amounts in most foods eaten away from home. It also is found in table salt and other seasonings. If your doctor wants you to cut back on sodium, try using herbs and spices instead of salt when you cook. **Limit canned, boxed or prepared meals, and fast foods.**

ALCOHOL

Alcohol is high in calories and has few nutrients. You may be able to have alcohol, but you should check with your doctor first. When you take insulin or certain diabetes pills, you are at risk for low blood sugar when you drink alcohol. Talk to your doctor about the effects of mixing alcohol with your medication. If your doctor says you can have alcohol once in awhile, follow these guidelines.

Drink alcohol with a meal. Alcohol can cloud your judgment and cause you to skip or delay a meal or snack, which can lead to low blood sugar. If your blood sugar is in good control, you may be able to include one or two servings of alcohol with a meal. One serving of alcohol may be a 4 oz. glass of dry wine, 12 oz. of lite beer, or 1 1/2 oz. of hard liquor (mixed with water or a sugar-free drink).

Avoid sweet drinks such as regular soda pop, fruit juice, liqueurs, sweet wine, and other drinks that are high in sugar or those made with tonic.

FIBER

Fiber is the part of foods, such as fruits, vegetables, and grains, that is not digested. Fiber does not add calories, but it does add bulk to your meal and helps you feel full longer. Fiber may be soluble or insoluble. Ask your dietitian how much fiber you should eat.

Soluble fiber

Soluble fiber may help lower blood sugar, especially after meals. Soluble fiber also may help lower cholesterol. Sources of soluble fiber are dried beans, peas, lentils, high-fiber cereals with oat bran or oatmeal, whole-grain breads, barley, and citrus fruits.

Insoluble fiber

Insoluble fiber is able to retain large amounts of water. It increases the volume of stool and makes it pass easily through the intestinal tract. Insoluble fiber may help prevent or treat constipation. Sources of insoluble fiber are wheat and corn bran, whole grains, some vegetables, and nuts.

EATING AWAY FROM HOME

- **Know your meal plan.** Know how many carbohydrate servings you are allowed for the meal you will eat.

- **Know your serving sizes.** Knowing what a serving looks like will help you judge serving sizes when you eat out.

- **Eat only the amount of food you should have.** You can always take the leftovers home with you. You may want to ask for a container *before* you begin eating. If the portion is larger than the serving size you should have, you can put the extra amount in the container to take home. That way you will be less likely to overeat.

- **Ask what is in the dish and how it is made.** Some foods have added sugars or are cooked in butter. Don't be afraid to ask for items that are not on the menu. Many restaurants will make special dishes or substitute one item for another.

- **Be careful when ordering fast food.** Many fast foods are high in saturated fat, cholesterol, and sodium.

- **Plan ahead.** If you take insulin, find out what time you will be eating. If you will be eating later than usual, eat a snack before you go. Be careful when taking insulin before you arrive at the restaurant. If the meal is delayed, you could experience low blood sugar. Talk to your doctor or diabetes educator about how to avoid this problem.

  Call ahead to see if there is a waiting list or if you can be seated on time. Make sure that the people you are eating with know that it is important for you to eat at the right time.

- **Order baked, broiled, grilled** (without fat), **or steamed foods** rather than fried foods or foods that are breaded or served with sauce. Order salad dressing on the side.

WEIGHT CONTROL

Maintaining a healthy weight helps your body make better use of insulin. For some people, losing 10 to 15 pounds improves how the body uses insulin and helps achieve normal blood sugar levels. **The combination of weight loss and exercise is the best way to improve blood sugar.** Before starting any weight loss program, ask your doctor for advice on achieving a healthy weight. As you change your eating habits and/or increase your activity, you may need to adjust your diabetes medications. Work with your doctor on this.

To lose weight and keep it off:

- **Keep a food diary.** You may think you know how much you are putting into your mouth, but you can't be sure unless you keep a diary. Write down what you eat, when you eat, and how much you eat. Keep track of your calories, carbohydrates, and fat grams.

- **Take smaller portions.** Select only the amount of meat or meat substitute on your meal plan. Switch to low-fat or fat-free salad dressing, mayonnaise, margarine, or butter. Weigh and measure food to help you with your portions.

- **Eat slowly.** Rapid eating may cause you to eat more food than you need. It takes 20 minutes for your stomach to tell your head that you are full. Put your fork down between bites. Sit down to eat. Don't eat while you are doing something else, such as watching TV or riding in a car.

- **Look for low-fat, low-sugar cookbooks** that will help you prepare healthy meals. Bake, broil, grill, or steam foods.

- **Combine regular exercise with changes in your diet.**

When you cut back on portions and increase your activity level, low blood sugar may occur. Talk to your healthcare team about making some changes that will help you prevent low blood sugar from occurring.

EXERCISE

Regular exercise can help:

- **Control your blood sugar.** Regular exercise helps insulin work better by allowing more sugar to enter your cells.

- **Control your weight.** Regular exercise burns extra calories and increases the rate at which your body burns calories.

- **Boost your energy.** When you exercise regularly, your heart can pump more blood through your body with less effort. This allows you to do more without getting tired.

- **Keep your heart and blood vessels healthy.** People with diabetes are at an increased risk for heart and blood vessel disease. Exercise reduces that risk.

Types of exercise

The best exercises for your heart, lungs, and blood vessels are **aerobic exercises**. They work large muscles non-stop for at least 20 to 30 minutes and gradually increase breathing and heart rates. Examples of aerobic exercises are jogging, brisk walking, biking, rowing, and swimming. If your health care team approves, you may want to add weight training to your workouts. Lifting weights helps you control your blood sugar. Weight lifting also builds muscle and helps you maintain a healthy weight.

Getting started

See your doctor for advice *before* you exercise. Certain complications may be aggravated by some types of exercise. People with an eye condition called retinopathy should also see an eye specialist before doing any type of exercise. If you take insulin, your food or insulin dose may need to be adjusted on physically active days. **If you are just beginning to exercise, start out slowly. Gradually increase your pace and the amount of time you exercise.**

By exercising, some people with Type 2 diabetes have been able to decrease or even eliminate the need for diabetes medication.

WARM UP AND COOL DOWN

Warm up for 5 to 10 minutes before your workout to get your body ready for your activity. Cool down for 5 to 10 minutes after your workout to bring your heart rate down. This helps prevent injuries to muscles and joints. You can warm up and cool down by walking or biking slowly for a few minutes.

Precautions

- **Check your blood sugar** before and after you exercise. If you plan to exercise for more than an hour, test your blood sugar during exercise as well.

- **Wear medical identification.**

- **Carry a mobile phone with you** in case you need help.

- **Don't exercise** if you are ill, if there are ketones in your urine, or if your blood sugar is above 240 or below 100 mg/dL.

- **Don't inject insulin into an area of your body that you will use during exercise.** For example, do not inject insulin into your legs if you will be riding a bike.

- **Watch for signs of low blood sugar.** If you don't usually have symptoms, check your blood sugar *during* exercise as well as before and after. (Low blood sugar can occur right after you exercise or it may be delayed. It can occur anytime up to 24 hours after you have exercised).

To prevent low blood sugar:

- **Take along a source of carbohydrate** in case of low blood sugar. One carbohydrate serving is 15 grams. Each of these examples contain 15 grams of carbohydrate: 3 square glucose tablets or 4 round glucose tablets; 2 pieces of hard candy; or 8 Lifesavers®.

- **Don't exercise when your insulin is working its hardest (peak).**

- **Eat a light carbohydrate snack about 30 minutes before you exercise** if your blood sugar is below 100 mg/dL, and you will be exercising at a moderate to high intensity.

More precautions

- **Have a medical exam before you begin** any type of exercise, especially if you:

  - have heart disease
  - are over 35
  - have high blood pressure
  - have high cholesterol
  - have a family history of heart disease

- **Tell your doctor about any unusual symptoms** you have during or after exercise, such as:

  - discomfort in your chest, neck, jaw, arms
  - nausea
  - dizziness or fainting
  - shortness of breath
  - short-term changes in vision

- **If you have diabetes complications,** ask your doctor about precautions.

People with numbness in their feet or legs should not run, jog, or walk long distances without a doctor's approval. People with eye problems should see an eye specialist before doing any type of exercise.

- **Don't exercise outdoors** when the weather is too hot and humid or too cold.

- **Wear the proper shoes.** Check your feet after you exercise. Treat any foot problems as soon as they appear.

INSULIN

You cannot live without insulin. If your body does not make enough insulin, you will need to take insulin. There is not one "right" insulin dose or way to take insulin. Each person must work with his or her doctor or diabetes educator to determine what is best. You must do what is necessary to keep your blood sugar within your target range.

The main kinds of insulin include:
- rapid-acting insulin (clear)
- fast-acting insulin (clear)
- medium-acting insulin (cloudy)
   NPH is the only cloudy insulin
- long-acting insulin (clear) – *Lantus & Levemir*
- a mix of fast- and medium-acting insulin (cloudy)

The types of insulin are different in these ways:
- onset – how soon they begin to work
- peak – when they are working the hardest
- duration – how long they keep working

How much insulin do you need? You need as much insulin as it takes to control your blood sugar. No one can tell you exactly how much that is, but your healthcare team will decide where to start. Sometimes it takes many adjustments to figure it out. **Some of the things that can affect your need for insulin are:**

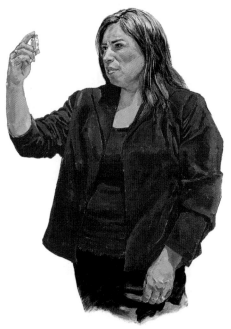

- how much you weigh
- how fit you are (how much fat and muscle you have)
- how sensitive your cells are to insulin
- how much you eat
- what kinds of foods you eat
- what other medications you take
- your emotions (such as stress)

Getting the right insulin dose is a lot like tailoring a suit. You might start with a suit right off the rack. Then the tailor nips and tucks until it is just right.

MORE ABOUT INSULIN

The chart below shows the average onset, peak, and duration of some insulins. If your insulin is not listed here, ask for information.

Insulin Type	Starts Working (onset)	Working the Hardest (peak)	How long it lasts (duration)
Rapid-acting Insulin			
Apidra (Glulisine)	5 to 15 min	55 min	3 to 4 hrs
Humalog (Lispro)	5 to 15 min	20 min to 1 1/2 hrs	3 to 4 hrs
Novolog (Aspart)	10 to 20 min	1 to 3 hrs	3 to 5 hrs
Fast-acting Insulin			
Regular	30 to 45 min	2 to 4 hrs	5 to 6 hrs
Medium-acting Insulin			
NPH	1 to 1 1/2 hrs	6 to 10 hrs	14 to 16 hrs
Long-acting Insulin			
Lantus (Glargine)	1 to 2 hrs	Flat	21 to 24 hrs
Levemir (Detemir)	1 to 2 hrs	Flat	24 hrs
Premixed Insulin			
70/30	30 min	2 to 6 hrs	10 to 16 hrs
Humalog Mix 50/50	30 min	2 to 6 hrs	10 to 16 hrs
Humalog Mix 75/25	5 to 15 min	1 to 4 hrs	10 to 16 hrs
Novolog Mix 70/30	20 min	2 to 4 hrs	Up to 24 hrs

The insulins Lantus and Levemir <u>cannot</u> be mixed with any other insulin. Each of these insulins must be given as a separate shot. Lantus and Levemir should be taken at approximately the same time of the day.

Pre-mixed insulin

Pre-mixed insulin is two kinds of insulin already mixed in one bottle. With pre-mixed insulin, you do not have to mix two kinds of insulins. The mixing is done for you. Many pre-mixed insulins come in insulin pens or cartridges. Ask your doctor for information on pre-mixed insulin.

Insulin pens or cartridges

Insulin pens or cartridges are easy to use. You simply screw the needle into the end of the pen, dial in the desired insulin dose, and then click down on a button to deliver the insulin. Some pens are disposable while others have replaceable insulin cartridges.

INSULIN PUMP

An insulin pump delivers a small amount of insulin continuously throughout the day and night. A needle is placed into the fatty tissue (usually in the abdomen). It stays in place for a few days. The needle is attached to tubing which connects to the pump. The pump is worn on a belt or placed in a pocket.

When you use an insulin pump you do not have to take insulin shots because the pump delivers the insulin you need. The insulin pump allows you to set a **basal rate** or background insulin, which is delivered continuously.

It also allows you to set a **bolus rate**, which is the insulin given when you eat a meal or when you have high blood sugar. You are able to tell the pump how many grams of carbohydrate you have eaten and what your blood sugar is at the present time. The pump will then determine how much insulin you need.

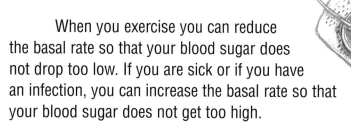

When you exercise you can reduce the basal rate so that your blood sugar does not drop too low. If you are sick or if you have an infection, you can increase the basal rate so that your blood sugar does not get too high.

Using an insulin pump is another way of managing your diabetes. **The insulin pump cannot control your blood sugar by itself. It requires commitment from you.** You must follow your meal plan and give your pump accurate information.

Even if you are using an insulin pump, you will still need to check your blood sugar on a regular basis. It is also important to follow your treatment guidelines and keep in touch with your healthcare team. If you have questions about your insulin pump, contact your diabetes educator, diabetes nurse, or healthcare provider.

TAKING INSULIN

Your insulin shot may be given with a syringe or with an insulin pen. If it is injected with a syringe, you must fill the syringe with insulin from a bottle. If you are using a pen, follow the instructions that come with the pen. Some pens are prefilled with the type of insulin you need—other pens may need a cartridge.

Insulin is measured in units. The number of units you take is your dose. Your dose is based on the amount of insulin you need to control your blood sugar. At first your dose may change often. Weight gain or loss, changes in diet or activities, or illness may affect the dose.

Insulin storage

You do not have to store your insulin bottle or pen in the refrigerator between injections. But you should store unopened insulin bottles or extra pen cartridges in the refrigerator. Injecting cold insulin can be uncomfortable. Insulin that has been refrigerated can be warmed by rolling the bottle or pen between your hands.

- **Keep your insulin away from very cold temperatures.** Insulin is good to use if it is stored (at room temperature or in a refrigerator) at a temperature between 36 and 86 degrees F. If you are traveling and are keeping your insulin in a cooler, make sure it does not freeze or come in contact with ice.

- **Keep your insulin away from hot temperatures or direct sunlight.** If the insulin gets too hot or too cold, it will not work as well and you may develop high blood sugar.

- **Check the expiration date on your insulin before you open it.** Throw away any outdated bottles of insulin.

- **Ask your diabetes educator how long you can use your insulin.**

Type of insulin	How long you can use it
Pens / Cartridges with cloudy insulin	14 days
Vials / Pens / Cartridges	28 days
Levemir	42 days

WHERE TO INJECT INSULIN

For insulin to be absorbed by your body, it should be injected into the fatty tissue just under your skin. The best places to inject insulin are the abdomen, buttocks, hips, thighs, and upper arms.

Different areas absorb insulin faster than others. Insulin enters the bloodstream fastest from the abdomen and more slowly from the buttocks. Your blood sugar may vary when different areas are used. Your doctor or diabetes nurse will help you decide which areas should be used for your injections.

CHANGING SITES

Repeated injections into the same spot can cause indentations, lumps, or a thickening in the skin. This makes it harder for insulin to be absorbed. For this reason, you will need to change the area (site) you use for your injection.

You may want to use one area of your body and change sites in that area. Sites should be about 1 inch apart. Do not inject too close to moles or scars. Depending on how many injections you need each day, your doctor may want you to use one area for a week or two before moving on to another area.

What you do after your shot can make a difference in how quickly insulin is absorbed. Parts of your body that are used during strenuous work or exercise will absorb insulin faster than other areas. For example, if you are going to use your arms and legs for strenuous work or exercise, your doctor or diabetes nurse may want you to use another site for your injection.

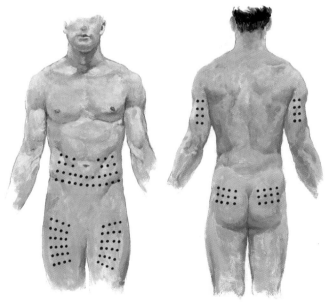

Keep your injection sites about 1" apart.

HOW TO DRAW UP ONE TYPE OF INSULIN

1. Wash your hands with soap and water. Check the label on the insulin bottle. Make sure it is the right type. Check the expiration date. Don't use outdated insulin.

2. Gently roll the bottle of insulin. Be sure the insulin is completely mixed. If the insulin is cloudy, always roll the bottle at least 20 times to make sure it is mixed well.

3. Wipe the top of the bottle with alcohol. Remove the needle cap from the syringe. Do not touch the needle.

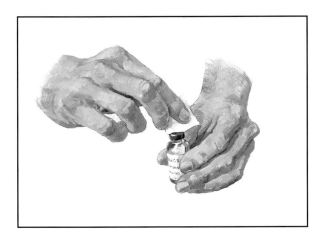

4. Fill the empty syringe with air equal to the amount of insulin you will take.

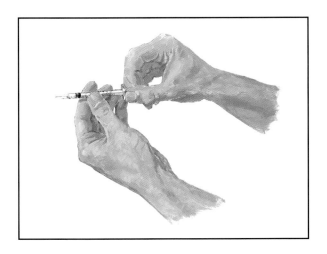

5. Push the needle into the bottle. Push the air from the syringe into the bottle. This makes it easier to draw out the insulin.

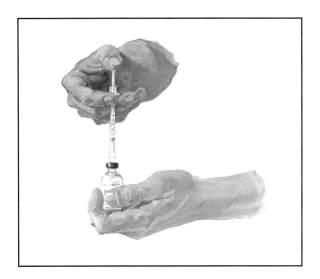

6. Keep the needle in the bottle. Turn the bottle upside down. Pull the plunger back. Fill the syringe with the number of units you need.

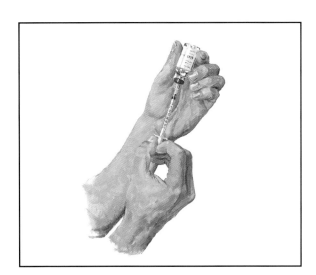

7. Look at the insulin in the syringe. If you see air bubbles, push the insulin back into the bottle and slowly draw it up again. Pull the needle out of the bottle. If you need to lay the syringe down before taking your injection, put the needle cap back on.

HOW TO INJECT INSULIN

1. Clean the injection site with soap and water or an alcohol swab. Let the area dry.

2. Remove the needle cover. Hold the syringe like a pencil. Gently pinch up a fold of skin.

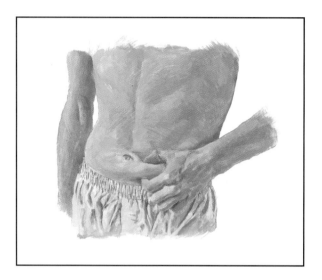

3. Position the needle at a 90 degree angle to the injection site (straight up and down). Insert the entire length of the needle into the fold of skin.

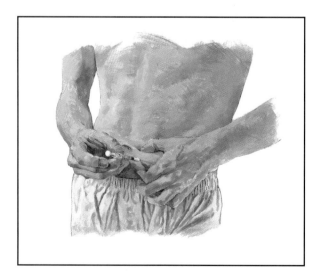

4. Let go of the pinched skin. Push the plunger all the way down.

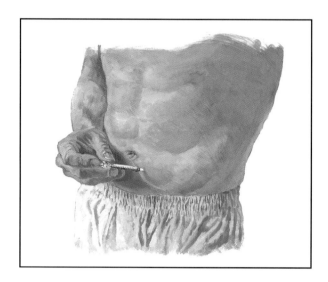

5. Once the insulin is injected, slowly count to 5 and pull the needle out. Place an alcohol wipe or cotton ball at the site and apply pressure. Do not massage the area.

6. Put your equipment in a covered, puncture-proof container. Mark it with "do not recycle" and throw it away.

Some areas of the country require that all syringes, needles, and lancets be destroyed. Check with your local waste authority if you have questions about equipment disposal.

If you have questions about injecting your insulin or about the type of insulin you are using, talk to your doctor or diabetes educator.

Do not change the amount of insulin you take without your doctor's approval.

HOW TO MIX TWO INSULINS

Your doctor may prescribe a mixed dose of fast-acting and medium-acting insulin for better blood sugar control. You will need to combine them in one syringe and take them as one injection.

You can identify the insulin by how it looks:

- rapid-acting and fast-acting insulins are **clear**
- medium-acting and long-acting insulins are **cloudy**
- long-acting *Lantus* and *Levemir* are **clear**

Note: Even though Lantus (Glargine) and Levemir (Detemir) are clear, they cannot be mixed with any other type of insulin.

1. Gently roll the *cloudy* bottle of insulin. Be sure the insulin is completely mixed.

2. Wipe off the tops of both insulin bottles with the same alcohol swab.

3. Remove the needle cap from the syringe. Do not touch the needle. Fill the empty syringe with air equal to the amount of **cloudy** insulin you will be taking.

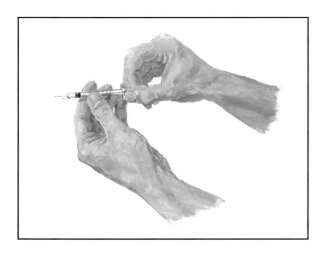

4. Inject the air from your syringe into the bottle of *cloudy* insulin.

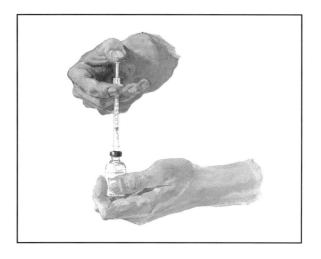

5. Do not draw up the *cloudy* insulin yet. Remove the needle from the bottle of **cloudy** insulin (syringe should be empty).

6. Fill your syringe with air equal to the amount of *clear* insulin you will be taking. Inject the air from your syringe into the bottle of **clear** insulin.

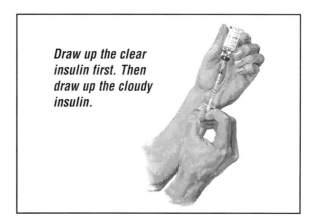

Draw up the clear insulin first. Then draw up the cloudy insulin.

7. Draw up the amount of *clear* insulin you will need. Remove air bubbles from the insulin. Now insert the needle back into the **cloudy** insulin. Draw up the amount of **cloudy** insulin you need.

Follow the steps on page 30 for your injection.

USING AN INSULIN PEN

If you are using medication that is injected with an insulin pen, follow these instructions or ask your healthcare team for information. You will need an insulin pen, pen needle, and an alcohol swab.

1. Wash your hands. Remove the cap from the pen and wipe the rubber stopper with an alcohol swab.

2. If the insulin in the pen is cloudy, *mix the insulin by gently moving the pen back and forth from top to bottom. Do this at least 20 times.* Repeat until the insulin appears uniformly white and cloudy.

3. Remove the protective tape from the pen needle and screw it onto the pre-filled pen. The first time you use the pen, turn the dose dial to *8 units.* Hold the pen with the needle pointing up. Tap the reservoir gently a few times.

4. Remove both the plastic outer cap and the needle cap. With the needle pointing up, press the button as far as it will go and see if a short stream of insulin is pushed out of the needle. If not, repeat the procedure until a short stream of insulin appears.

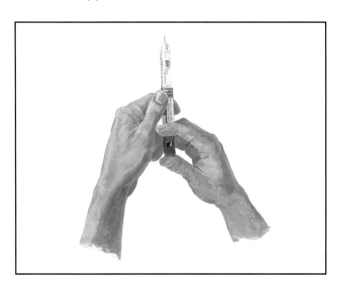

5. Make sure the dose selector is set at zero. Dial the dose selector to 1 and with the needle pointed up, press the button and make sure a drop of insulin comes out. Make sure the dose selector is back to zero.

6. Dial the the number of units of insulin you need to inject. If you passed the number of units you need, the dose can be corrected by dialing back and forth.

7. Choose your injection site. Pinch the skin at the injection site and push the needle into the skin fold. Push the button all the way in.

8. With the button pushed all the way in, keep the needle in the skin for at least the slow count of 5 to ensure that the full dose of insulin has been delivered.

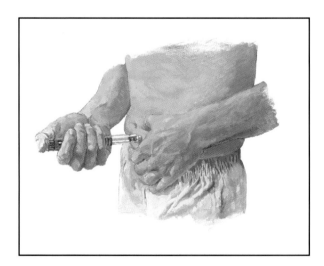

9. Keep the button pushed in until the needle is withdrawn from the skin. Carefully recap the needle and place the pen in storage.

ORAL DIABETES MEDICATIONS (PILLS)

If meal planning, exercise, and weight loss do not lower blood sugar (for a person with Type 2 diabetes), your doctor may want you to take a diabetes pill. This type of medication is not insulin. Some pills are taken together. Others may be taken along with insulin.

Some diabetes pills may lower your blood sugar too much. Be sure to watch for signs of low blood sugar. If low blood sugar occurs often, tell your doctor. Your medication may need to be adjusted.

Trade Name	Generic Name	How it works	Possible side effects
Micronase	Glyburide	Causes the pancreas to make more insulin	Low blood sugar. Allergy to sulfa
Diabeta			
Glynase			
Glucotrol	Glipizide	Causes the pancreas to make more insulin	Low blood sugar. Allergy to sulfa
Glucotrol XL			
Amaryl	Glimepride		
Prandin	Repaglinide	Causes the pancreas to make more insulin	Low blood sugar
Starlix	Nateglinide		
Glucophage	Metformin	Helps the body make better use of insulin	Gastrointestinal disturbances
Glucophage XR			
Glumetza			
Fortamet			
Riomet (liquid form)			
Precose	Acarbose	Slows the digestion of carbohydrate foods	Gastrointestinal disturbances
Glyset	Miglitol		
Avandia	Rosiglitazone	Helps the body make better use of insulin	May cause swelling in the feet or hands. Monitor with liver function tests.
Actos	Pioglitazone		

Combinations: A combination medication may be prescribed. A combination medication is two diabetes medications in one pill. They can have the benefits and side-effect of each one of the pills in the combination. Examples of such medications are Avandamet, Glucovance, Metaglip, Actoplus Met, and Avandaryl. Avandamet is a combination of Avandia and Metformin. Glucovance is a combination of Glyburide and Metformin. Metaglip is a combination of Glipizide and Metformin. Actoplus Met is a combination of Actos and Metformin. Avandaryl is a combination of Avandia and Amaryl. Duetact is a combination of Actos and Amaryl.

Tell your doctor about all the medications you take. Certain medications (even over-the-counter or herbal medications) can affect the way your diabetes pills work. Talk to your doctor before you drink alcohol. Certain diabetes pills, when mixed with alcohol, may cause nausea, dizziness, or a rapid heartbeat.

OTHER DIABETES MEDICATIONS

New medications are now available. These medications are not insulin, but they do work with insulin to give people with diabetes more stable blood sugar levels.

Injectable Medications	Oral Medications (pills)
Symlin (Pramlintide)	Januvia
Byetta (Evenatide)	Januvamet

Symlin

Symlin (Pramlintide) is used with insulin to lower blood sugar, especially high blood sugar that happens after meals. Symlin comes in a pre-filled pen with fixed dosing. It can be used with both Type 1 and Type 2 diabetes. Symlin is given at mealtimes. Symlin does not replace daily insulin, but it may lower the amount of insulin you need, especially before meals.

Even when Symlin is carefully added to your mealtime insulin therapy, your blood sugar may drop too low. If low blood sugar happens, it usually occurs within 3 hours after a Symlin injection. That's why it is important for you and your family and friends to know how to recognize and treat low blood sugar.

Guidelines for taking Symlin:

- **Symlin should be refrigerated up to the first dose.** Then it may be stored at room temperature not to exceed 86 degrees F.

- **Do not use Symlin if you are not going to eat or if you are eating only a small meal** containing less than 250 calories or 30 grams of carbohydrate.

- **Do not use Symlin if you are sick or having a medical procedure** and cannot eat your meal.

- **If you miss or forget a dose of Symlin,** wait until the next meal and take your usual dose.

Keep careful records of your blood sugar levels, your insulin use, and changes in your weight.

Byetta

Byetta (Evenatide) was developed to help treat people with Type 2 diabetes in a different way than pills or insulin. Byetta helps your body produce the right amount of insulin at the right time and stops your liver from producing too much glucose (blood sugar) after meals. Byetta also reduces appetite and slows down how quickly food and glucose leave the stomach, helping to prevent high blood sugar after you eat.

Byetta is taken as an injection, twice a day, at any time within the 60 minutes before the morning and evening meals. Byetta should not be taken after a meal. Byetta comes in a prefilled pen with fixed dosing. It may be used with metformin, or a sulfonylurea or a thiazonlidinedione medication, or both.

Guidelines for taking Byetta:

- If a dose is missed, wait until the next scheduled dose and take only the prescribed dose at that time.

- After the first use, Byetta can be stored at room temperature not to exceed 77 degrees F. Store any unopened Byetta in the refrigerator. Do not allow Byetta to freeze.

When Byetta is used with a medication that contains a sulfonylurea, low blood sugar is a possible side effect. The dose of your sulfonylurea medication may need to be reduced while you use Byetta. If your doctor has prescribed Byetta, it is very important for you to know the symptoms of low blood sugar and know how to treat it.

Nausea is common when first starting Byetta, but it usually decreases over time. Talk with your doctor or diabetes nurse about any side effects you experience.

Januvia

Januvia (Sitagliptin) is a medication which helps lower blood sugar levels in people with Type 2 diabetes. It is taken once a day. Januvia helps keep blood sugar levels balanced, especially after you eat. It also reduces the amount of sugar made by your liver after you eat, when your body does not need it. Talk to your diabetes nurse or educator if you are taking other medications with Januvia, or if you have any questions about this medication. Also available is a Januvamet, which is a combination of Januvia and Metformin.

TESTING FOR CONTROL

Your doctor will do blood tests from time to time to see if your meal plan, exercise, and medications are working together to control your diabetes.

A **single blood glucose test** shows your blood sugar level at the exact time it is taken. In this test, blood is drawn and measured before or after a meal. Since blood sugar can vary over the course of a day, a single blood glucose test is not the best way to check for *overall* control.

An **A1c test** show an average of your blood sugar over the past 3 months. Performing this test is a good way to check *overall* control. For someone who does not have diabetes, the level of A1c is usually between 4 and 6 percent. These levels may vary depending on the laboratory that performs the test. When diabetes is poorly controlled, A1c may be 8 percent or higher. According to the *American Diabetes Association,* your goal should be to keep your A1c level at 7 percent or below (which is equal to a blood sugar level of 150 mg/dL).

Why is knowing your A1c number important?

Research has found a link between high blood sugar levels and diabetes complications. Reducing your blood sugar to near normal levels can help reduce your risk of eye problems by up to 76%; nerve damage up to 60%; and severe kidney problems up to 56%.

The result of an A1c test cannot be changed by a day or two, or even a week of changes in your blood sugar. It can only be changed by weeks of careful attention to your meal plan, exercise, and medication.

Between visits to your doctor, you will need to check your own blood sugar. This is called **self blood monitoring.** Doing this is useful for finding out how high or low your blood sugar is at key times of the day such as first thing in the morning before you eat; before a meal or 2 hours after a meal; before or after exercise; and at bedtime or occasionally in the middle of the night.

MONITORING YOUR BLOOD SUGAR

Self blood monitoring is done by pricking your finger and putting the blood on or next to a test strip. Self blood monitoring is not just for people who take medication. Even if you don't take any diabetes medication, checking your blood sugar shows you whether diet and exercise alone are working to control your blood sugar. Self blood monitoring lets you make changes in your diabetes management plan that will keep your blood sugar as close to normal as possible.

From testing your blood sugar you can tell:

- what your blood sugar level is at the moment
- how food, exercise, medications, stress, or illness are affecting your blood sugar
- if you have signs of very low or very high blood sugar

When should you check your blood sugar?

If you've just been diagnosed or if you are starting a new medication, you may be asked to test more often. Once you've settled into a plan, the frequency may change. You will be told how often to check your blood sugar and what your target blood sugar range should be.

SELF BLOOD MONITORING

To test your blood sugar, a test strip is inserted into a machine called a **blood glucose meter**. A small drop of blood is placed on or next to the test strip. The meter reads the strip and shows the results of the test through a display window.

Before you test your blood sugar, clean your finger with soap and water or an alcohol swab. Let your finger dry. Prick the side of your finger (using this area will be less painful). If you have trouble getting blood, wash your finger with warm water. Hold your hand down or squeeze your finger. Some meters allow you to poke your forearm, stomach, or thigh to get a drop of blood. If you think you have high or low blood sugar, you should only use blood from your finger to test your blood sugar.

RECORD KEEPING

Changes in your food, work, and exercise can affect your diabetes. Recording this information shows you and your health care team how well your blood sugar is being controlled. It also shows how changes in your daily habits can affect your blood sugar. Bring your records along when you see your doctor or diabetes educator.

Another reason to record your blood sugar is to look for blood sugar patterns. For example, there may be times when your blood sugar is always high or always low. A pattern like this may be a sign that your medication (insulin or pills) may need to be adjusted. Your doctor or diabetes educator will help you look for patterns in your daily diabetes records.

Date	Breakfast	After Breakfast	Lunch	After Lunch	Dinner	After Dinner	Bedtime	Comments (diet, stress, exercise, illness, etc.)

LOW BLOOD SUGAR

When you take insulin or other diabetes medication, it is possible for your blood sugar to drop too low. Normally, a blood sugar below 70 mg/dL is considered too low. **Low blood sugar** is sometimes called an insulin reaction. Most people with diabetes have low blood sugar at one time or another.

Low blood sugar might occur if:

- you miss or delay a meal or eat less than usual
- you are more physically active than usual
- you take too much insulin or other diabetes medication

Early warning signs:

- hunger
- headache
- sweaty or clammy feeling
- dizziness or shaky feeling
- faster than normal heartbeat
- confusion
- nervousness or irritability
- numbness or tingling around the mouth or lips

If low blood sugar is not treated right away, it can lead to seizures, unconsciousness, or coma. If low blood sugar occurs more than twice a week, tell your doctor or diabetes nurse.

HOW TO TREAT LOW BLOOD SUGAR

If you are conscious and able to swallow, you should eat or drink 15 grams of carbohydrate. Each of these examples contain 15 grams of carbohydrate:

- 3 square glucose tablets or 4 round glucose tablets
- 1/2 cup of fruit juice or regular soft drink
- 8 Lifesavers® or 2 pieces of hard candy
- 1 tablespoon of sugar, honey, or syrup
- 8 ounces of milk

Wait 15 minutes. If the symptoms have not gone away, eat or drink another serving from this list. If you still do not feel better, call someone to help you. If your meal is more than 30 minutes away, you should eat a snack with carbohydrate and protein, such as 1/2 of a sandwich, or crackers and peanut butter or cheese.

Know how to give a
glucagon injection

It is a good idea for your
family members, close
friends, and co-workers
to know how to give a
glucagon injection.

Here are some general
guidelines for the person
who may be giving your
injection:

- **Read the instructions
  that come with the
  glucagon kit.** The
  instructions will tell you
  how to prepare the
  injection.

- **Place your loved one on
  his or her side.**

- **Use the steps on page
  30** to inject the glucagon.

- **After the injection,
  check your loved one.**
  He or she should start to
  feel better. When your
  loved one is able, give
  him or her a healthy
  snack.

- **If your loved one does
  not respond to the
  injection,** call 911 or
  your local emergency
  number.

- **Be sure to check the
  expiration date** on the
  glucagon kit.

Have your family review
the instructions that come
with your glucagon kit
regularly.

SEVERE LOW BLOOD SUGAR

If the symptoms of low blood sugar become severe or you
are unable to swallow, call 911 (or your local emergency number)
or have someone take you to the nearest emergency room for
treatment. Your family may be taught to give **glucagon**, a drug that
increases blood sugar. It comes in a kit with a syringe and
instructions on how to use the drug. Ask your doctor for more
information on glucagon.

How to prevent low blood sugar:

- **Be consistent about the amount and timing of meals,** snacks,
  and medication. Your food intake must balance with the insulin
  working in your body.

- **Don't skip meals or snacks.** Always eat on time.

- **Measure your medication carefully.** Take the exact amount of
  medication you need and take it on time.

- **Plan ahead.** If you know you are going to be more active, adjust
  your medication or eat additional snacks. Adjustments you make
  will depend on the results of your blood tests and the type of
  activity you do.

- **Record low blood sugar reactions.** Show the records to your
  health care team so they can see patterns that are causing your
  reactions and help you prevent them.

- **Always carry a quick source of carbohydrate** in case you have
  low blood sugar.

- **Once your blood sugar is above 70, check the timing of your
  next meal or snack.** If your next meal is more than 1 hour away,
  eat a snack right away.

    The snack should be 1 carbohydrate and 1 meat, such as:

    - 1/2 of a sandwich
    - 4 to 6 crackers and 1 ounce of cheese.

HIGH BLOOD SUGAR

High blood sugar is any number above your target blood sugar range, which for many people is 90 to 130 mg/dL before meals. High blood sugar can occur for many reasons such as lack of exercise, skipping your medication or not taking the right amount, stress, illness, overeating or not following your meal plan.

Because high blood sugar happens gradually, the signs are not always easy to notice.

If you have high blood sugar, you may:

- feel very thirsty
- have to go to the bathroom often
- feel very tired or weak
- have blurred vision or problems seeing
- have vaginal or genital itching

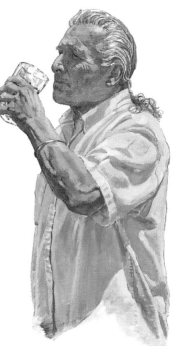

How to treat high blood sugar

- adjust your medication if your doctor or your diabetes nurse tells you to do so
- test your blood sugar every couple of hours
- test your urine for ketones if your blood sugar is over 240 mg/dL (for Type 1 diabetes only)
- follow your diabetes meal plan
- drink fluids - at least 8 ounces every hour

Feeling very thirsty may be a sign of high blood sugar.

Call your doctor right away if:

- your urine ketones show moderate or large amounts, or you have 2 positive tests
- your blood sugar is more than 240 mg/dL twice in a row

To prevent high blood sugar, follow your meal plan, exercise program, and medication instructions. Check your blood sugar often. Never stop taking your diabetes medication without your doctor's OK.

TESTING FOR KETONES (for Type 1 diabetes only)

If there is not enough insulin in your body to use sugar for energy, stored fat is broken down and used. When fat is used for energy instead of sugar, harmful acids called ketones form. Ketones build up in the blood and eventually spill into the urine. The buildup of ketones can lead to a serious condition called ketoacidosis. If it is not treated right away, ketoacidosis can lead to a coma or even death.

A urine test is used to check for ketones. Always have products on hand to test your urine.

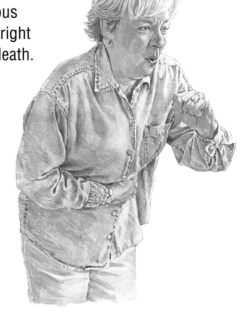

Test your urine for ketones IF:

- your blood tests are 240 mg/dL or higher
- you are sick or you have an infection
- you are under a lot of stress
- you have lost weight and you don't know why
- you do not feel well, even if your blood sugar is in the normal range or low

When you are sick, check your urine for ketones.

Call your doctor if your blood sugar is above 240 mg/dL twice in a row and there are ketones in your urine. You will be told what to do and whether to take more insulin. If you are not able to drink fluids, your doctor may want you to go to the hospital for treatment.

Signs of ketoacidosis:

- nausea and/or abdominal pain or cramping
- flushed skin
- sweet, fruity odor to your breath
- rapid breathing
- loss of appetite
- unconsciousness
- symptoms of high blood sugar (see page 41)

It is not enough for you alone to know about ketoacidosis. Those close to you should also be aware of the warning signs.

CARE DURING ILLNESS

When you are sick, diabetes is harder to control. Even a cold can cause your diabetes to go out of control. If you have Type 1 diabetes and your blood sugar stays too high, ketones can appear in your urine and ketoacidosis can occur. High blood sugar, along with sweating, vomiting, or diarrhea can lead to extra fluid loss.

- Take your insulin or diabetes pills even if you don't feel like eating. Ask your doctor how much to take. During illness you may need more medication than usual.

- Test your blood sugar often. You may need to test your blood sugar every 2 to 4 hours. Test often until you feel better and/or your blood sugar returns to normal.

- Call your doctor if your blood sugar is greater than 240 mg/dL for 2 tests in a row, or if your urine ketones are moderate or high.

- Try to eat foods from your meal plan and drink about 1/2 to 1 cup of fluid every 30 to 60 minutes. If you are able to eat as you usually do, you may try replacing water with a diet soft drink, club soda, or tea without sugar.

Call your doctor if you have:

- severe diarrhea or vomiting that lasts 6 to 12 hours or longer

- urine ketones in moderate or high amounts

- blood sugar greater than 240 mg/dL twice in a row

- fever greater than 100 degrees F for 24 to 48 hours

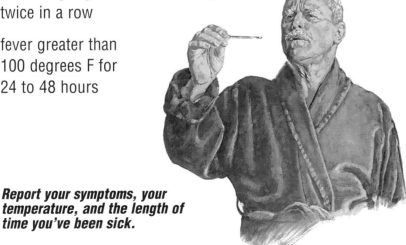

Report your symptoms, your temperature, and the length of time you've been sick.

Take Care of Yourself

- **Do *not* stop taking your insulin or diabetes pills** just because you are not eating as much as usual. You may need more of your medication during sick days. Taking no medication could result in a hospital stay.

- **Make a list of the over-the-counter medications you use.** Talk to your doctor or diabetes nurse about which items may affect your blood sugar.

  Some medications such as cold and flu remedies, or sore throat lozenges contain sugar. If your doctor tells you it is ok to take some of these medications, look for sugar-free products.

- **Keep appropriate medications on hand.** That way you won't take something inappropriate when you are ill or when someone else is taking care of you.

- **When you call your doctor, report:**
  - your symptoms
  - your temperature
  - length of time you've been sick
  - which over-the-counter medications you are taking
  - which herbal or alternative medications you are taking
  - whether you have been eating or drinking according to your usual meal plan
  - your blood sugar levels
  - your ketone levels

FOODS RECOMMENDED ON SICK DAYS

When you are sick, your doctor, diabetes educator, or your dietitian may suggest a liquid or semi-liquid diet. Follow your individual guidelines. Here are some suggestions:

Fruit

Choose one of these foods for every fruit on your meal plan (each item contains **15 grams of carbohydrate or 1 serving or choice**)

3/4 c. regular ginger ale	1 1/2 c. Gatorade®
1/3 c. grape juice	1/2 c. Kool-aid®
1/3 c. cranberry juice	1/2 c. lemonade
3 tsp. syrup or sugar	1/2 c. 7-up®
Popsicle (1 single bar or 1/2 of a twin bar)	1/2 c. apple juice

Milk

Choose one of these foods for every milk on your meal plan (each item contains **12 grams of carbohydrate or 1 serving or choice**)

1 c. milk	1/2 c. regular cocoa
1/4 c. custard	1 c. cream soup

Starch

Choose one of these foods for every starch on your meal plan (each item contains **15 grams of carbohydrate or 1 serving or choice**)

1/2 c. regular pudding	1/3 c. regular gelatin
1/2 c. ice cream	6 saltine crackers
1 c. chicken noodle soup	
1/2 c. cooked cereal	
1/4 c. sherbet	

A clear liquid diet may be suggested. This includes fat-free broth, consommé, and foods listed under fruit. You may need 15 to 20 servings spaced over the course of a day.

Do not have milk, milk products, and solid foods while you are on a clear liquid diet. If clear liquids agree with you, try the foods listed under milk and starch.

MEDICAL IDENTIFICATION

It's a good idea to wear medical identification. Should you be injured, your ID will let people know you have diabetes. One type of identification is called Medic Alert. It is recognized worldwide as identification of a health problem. A bracelet or necklace can be purchased which lists your medical condition as well as a 24-hour emergency number. Ask your healthcare team where to get medical identification or contact Medic Alert International at 1-(800) 432-5378 or www.medicalert.org

PREVENTING COMPLICATIONS

Complications may happen after someone has had diabetes for many years. Controlling blood sugar can delay or prevent many complications. While health problems can occur even if your diabetes is in good control, you will have a better chance of preventing problems if you know what to watch for.

Nerves

People with diabetes can develop nerve damage called neuropathy. Many areas of the body, such as the bladder, bowels, and other organs, can be affected. Symptoms include numbness, tingling, burning, or aching mainly in the feet, lower legs, and hands. It also can cause a loss of feeling. A person with nerve damage may not feel the pain of a sore. Controlling your blood sugar may help prevent neuropathy. If damage occurs, controlling your blood sugar may improve the function of damaged nerves.

Sexual problems

Usually, people with diabetes are able to perform sexual activities normally. However, in both men and women with diabetes, some problems can occur due to nerve damage and poor circulation. Men may suffer from impotence (inability to have or maintain an erection). Women may have a decrease in vaginal lubrication or an inability to reach orgasm. Sexual problems are not always permanent. They may be caused by stress, medication, or a change in hormone levels. For men, impotence may occur during a short period of high blood sugar, then go away once blood sugar levels return to normal. Talk to your doctor about any problems you are having. He or she can determine the cause and discuss treatment with you.

FEET

Loss of sensation in the feet due to nerve damage is a problem for people with diabetes. When this happens, you cannot rely on feelings of pain or extremes in temperature to warn you of problems. Poor circulation also may cause injuries to heal slowly or not at all.

To protect your feet:

- **Check your feet each day** for cuts, scratches, blisters, sores, or bruises. Call your doctor right away if you have:

    - an open sore on your foot
    - any infection in a cut or blister
    - a red, tender toe – possibly an ingrown toenail
    - any change in feeling – pain, tingling, or numbness
    - any puncture wound, such as if you step on a nail

- **Wash your feet each day** with warm water and mild soap. Test the water temperature with your inner arm before you wash your feet. Do not soak you feet. After washing your feet, dry them thoroughly, especially between the toes. Use a moisturizing cream to soften dry skin.

- **Cut your nails straight** across to prevent ingrown toenails. Do not trim corns or calluses or use iodine, peroxide, or strong antiseptics on your feet.

- **Protect your toes, feet, and legs.** Wear shoes that fit well. Shoes that are too tight can cut off circulation. Shoes that are too loose or rub can cause blisters or sores. Look inside and shake out your shoes and socks before putting them on your feet. Don't go barefoot. Wear protective shoes when you are at home, swimming, or on a beach.

- **Wear loose-fitting socks** if your feet are cold. Do not use hot water bottles or heating pads to warm your feet.

- **Have your feet checked each time you see your doctor.**

EYES

Diabetes can affect your eyes in many ways. In some cases, changes such as blurred vision may be temporary and can be helped by better diabetes control. But if diabetes has been present for a long time, it can cause changes in your eyes that threaten your vision. Some of the most common problems are listed here.

Cataracts

Cataracts are a gradual clouding of the lens of the eye. They reduce vision by preventing light from getting in. Surgery may be needed to correct the problem.

Glaucoma

Glaucoma is a common problem caused by the buildup of pressure in the eye, which is harmful to the nerves. Sometimes the pressure can be reduced with medication or surgery.

Retinopathy

Retinopathy is the result of changes in the retina, the tissue at the back of the eye that changes light into visual image. It is one of the most common causes of blindness. There are a number of treatments for retinopathy that can help prevent blindness or minimize the loss of vision.

High blood pressure also may contribute to retinopathy. Controlling your blood pressure, keeping your blood sugar close to normal, and having annual eye exams will help safeguard your vision.

See an eye specialist (ophthalmologist or optometrist) **once a year for a complete exam**. Your eye exam should include dilating your pupils so your doctor can look at the retina.

Call your eye specialist right away if you have sudden blurred vision, black spots, lines, or flashing lights in your field of vision.

Write down any questions you have and discuss them with your doctor, diabetes nurse, or diabetes educator.

HEART AND BLOOD VESSELS

Diabetes can damage the blood vessels that lead to the heart, brain, and legs. Scars can form inside blood vessels making them hard and rough. Fatty substances in the blood can stick to the rough lining inside the blood vessels. In time, blood vessels can become blocked and blood flow is restricted. A heart attack, stroke, or loss of circulation to the legs can occur.

To keep your heart and blood vessels healthy:

- **Keep your blood sugar in good control.** Check your blood sugar often and follow your treatment program.

- **Control your cholesterol.** Eating too much saturated fat, trans fat, and cholesterol can cause high blood cholesterol. When there is too much cholesterol in the blood, the extra amount builds up inside the arteries in the form of fatty deposits. Fatty deposits can block arteries and lead to a heart attack or stroke. Eat foods that are low in saturated fats, trans fats, and cholesterol.

- **Maintain a healthy weight.** Being overweight makes your heart work harder. People who are overweight are also more likely to have high blood pressure and high cholesterol.

- **Control your blood pressure.** High blood pressure damages blood vessels. People with diabetes are more likely to have high blood pressure than people who do not have diabetes. Have your blood pressure checked regularly. If it's high, follow the treatment your doctor recommends.

- **Don't use tobacco.** Tobacco narrows blood vessels and increases your risk of heart disease.

Teeth and gums

Dental problems tend to be more serious when diabetes is present. You can prevent tooth decay and periodontal disease (a disease caused by food collecting around the teeth and gums) by brushing your teeth every day. Floss every day to remove food your toothbrush can't reach. Have your teeth cleaned every 6 months. See your dentist if you have unusual pain, swelling, or excessive bleeding.

If you have trouble quitting, consider joining a stop-smoking program

KIDNEYS

People with diabetes are at risk for developing kidney disease. The kidneys help keep the right fluid balance in the body by filtering waste products from the blood. With kidney disease, the kidneys are unable to filter all the waste products from the body. This disease happens slowly, so it's possible to have it and not know it until the kidneys are already damaged.

To prevent kidney disease:

- **Control your blood sugar and your blood pressure.**

- **See your doctor once a year to check your kidneys.** Have a urine test (urinalysis) for microalbumin and/or a blood test for creatinine.

- **Treat bladder or urinary tract infections right away.** Symptoms include fever or chills; frequent urination or burning sensation when urinating; blood in the urine or cloudy, foul smelling urine; low back pain.

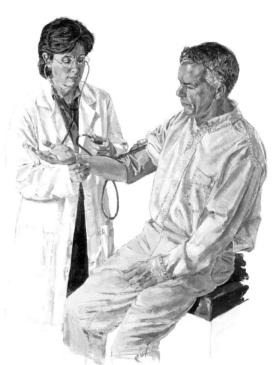

SKIN CARE

Treat bacterial infections as soon as you notice any of the symptoms. A bacterial infection can develop quickly from a minor injury. Infections caused by fungus are also a problem. Women may be bothered by vaginal yeast infections; in men, the genitals may become infected. Infected areas are usually red, inflamed, and itchy. See your doctor if you have these symptoms.

To keep your skin healthy, bathe or shower daily. Use a lanolin-based lotion to prevent dry skin. Dry your skin thoroughly. Apply talcum powder between skin folds. Wear cotton underwear. Change your underwear and stockings each day. To avoid fungus, wear slippers when using a public locker room or shower.

Treat small cuts, broken skin, or insect bites promptly. Clean your skin with mild soap and water. Do not soak the area. Cover it with a bandage. If the area has not started to heal within 48 hours, or if you notice redness or swelling, see your doctor right away.

Guidelines for taking your medications

- **When your doctor suggests a new medication,** ask how the drug will affect your diabetes and other health problems. Ask if the drug can be taken with other medications.

- **Keep a list of all the prescription and non-prescription medications you take** including herbal supplements and vitamins.

- **Every so often, review with your doctor all the medications** you take. A review is a good way to make sure you are taking the medications that are right for you.

- **Buy a drug reference book that lists** what the drug is for and possible side effects or interactions. Being well informed will help you be a better partner with your doctor.

- **Never take more or less medication** than your doctor told you to take. Never stop taking your medication without your doctor's OK.

- **If you forget to take your medication,** DO NOT double up on your next dose. Ask your doctor what to do.

- **Read labels carefully.** If you wear glasses, put them on. If the room is dark, turn on a light. Don't take your pills in the dark.

LIVING WITH DIABETES

Medications

Make sure you understand how and when to take your medication. Never change the dose or the way you take your medication without your doctor's approval.

Make a list of your prescription and non-prescription medications. Bring the list along when you see any of your healthcare providers. Your list should include things like cold and allergy medication, vitamins, and herbal remedies. If you have questions about any of your medications, discuss them with your doctor and your pharmacist. Report any medication side effects to your doctor right away.

Work

Your diabetes should not prevent you from working. Having diabetes or other health problems may make it unwise to choose certain types of jobs for safety or other reasons.

Type 1 diabetes is considered a disability under a special law called the Americans with Disabilities Act. This law protects all people with disabilities. It ensures that you cannot be discriminated against for most jobs because you have diabetes.

It's a good idea to tell your employer you have diabetes in case you have to adjust your schedule for meals or visits to the doctor. Also, let your co-workers know about your diabetes. Make sure they know what to do in case of an emergency. Provide emergency contacts including family members and healthcare professionals.

TRAVEL

By planning ahead you should be able to take trips. These suggestions can make traveling safe and enjoyable.

If you take insulin and plan to cross time zones, ask your doctor, nurse, or diabetes educator how to adjust your medication. Pack extra supplies. Put them in the bags you keep with you.

Check your blood sugar more often so you know how changes in your diet, exercise, and sleep affect you. Always carry fast-acting carbohydrates with you in case you have low blood sugar. Also carry some carbohydrate and protein foods for unexpected delays in your meal schedule.

If you travel by car, stop every couple of hours. Walk for a few minutes to improve blood flow. If you plan to get more exercise than usual during your trip, adjust your medication and food intake.

If you travel by plane, carry the diabetes supplies you need with you. Your insulin and blood testing strips should be kept with you and not placed in your general luggage. Bring them in the original box with the pharmacy label attached which tells the name of the medication or supply and your name. All lancets must be capped and enclosed with the glucose monitor.

Check with the airline before you go to be sure of their policy. Make sure you understand how to pack your supplies so that you will not have problems when you prepare to board your flight.

If you are traveling outside the United States, have any immunizations (shots) you need a few weeks before you go.

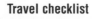

Travel checklist

- **Carry more medications and monitoring supplies** than you may need for the number of days in your trip.

- **Pack your medications and supplies** in your carry-on luggage.

- **Pack snacks for the ride to account for a delay** or sudden change in plans.

- **Plan your insulin doses for time in transit** in advance. Ask your diabetes educator how to adjust your medication for changes in time zones.

- **Monitor.** It's the only way you'll know how your travel and activities are affecting your blood sugar.

- **Stay hydrated.** Drink plenty of non-alcoholic, caffeine-free beverages.

- **Wear sunscreen** with an SPF of 30 or higher.

- **Never walk barefoot,** even on the beach. Always wear a protective shoe with a closed toe. Check your feet each day for cuts, sores, or blisters.

- **Ask your doctor to write a letter** on letterhead stationery explaining anything that another physician would need to know to care for you. The letter also may come in handy in case you are questioned about medications or equipment you are carrying.

PREGNANCY

With planning and good control, a woman who does not have diabetes complications has about the same chance of having a successful pregnancy as a woman without diabetes.

Changes that occur with pregnancy make it harder to control blood sugar. Your blood sugar should be as close to normal as possible before and during pregnancy. See your doctor often and check your blood sugar more frequently.

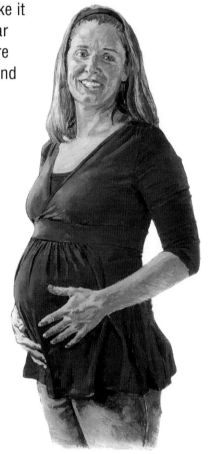

A woman who does not have diabetes can develop diabetes during pregnancy. Gestational diabetes usually appears in the 24th to 28th week of pregnancy. A balanced meal plan can help your body make better use of the insulin you have. If your blood sugar cannot be lowered by your meal plan, you will need insulin.

Gestational diabetes may go away after the baby is born, but it may reappear in future pregnancies. Women who have had gestational diabetes are at a greater risk for developing Type 2 diabetes later in life. Making healthy lifestyle changes is important during and after pregnancy.

KEEP LEARNING

Advances in diabetes care are happening all the time. Keep aware of them by checking with your diabetes educator on a regular basis. Learn as much as you can. Ask your doctor what routine tests you need for your eyes, feet, kidneys, and blood sugar. Take diabetes education classes at your local hospital or clinic.

Your attitude can make a big difference in how diabetes affects you. Diabetes can't be cured, but it can be controlled. How well your diabetes is controlled is up to you. Empower yourself, take charge, and you will control your diabetes instead of letting it control you.